The Negative Calorie Diet

Lose Weight and Burn More Calories Than You Consume With These Negative Calorie Foods

monetary loss due to the information herein, either directly or indirectly.

Respective authors own all copyrights not held by the publisher.

The information herein is offered for informational purposes solely, and is universal as so. The presentation of the information is without contract or any type of guarantee assurance.

The trademarks that are used are without any consent, and the publication of the trademark is without permission or backing by the trademark owner. All trademarks and brands within this book are for clarifying purposes only and are the owned by the owners themselves, not affiliated with this document.

Introduction

I want to thank you and congratulate you for purchasing the book, *"The Negative Calorie Diet - Lose Weight and Burn More Calories Than You Consume With These Negative Calorie Foods".*

This book looks at the negative calorie diet comprehensively and how you can lose weight while on the diet.

You probably know that foods such as tea and water have zero calories. However, have your heard about negative calorie foods? My guess would be that you have. While some foods are very low in calories, in truth, no food has negative calories. The concept of a negative calorie diet draws its belief from the fact that some foods require more energy to metabolize than the energy/calories they inject into your metabolism. Take for instance water or other succulent veggies like celery; the body requires fuel to break them down and excrete their waste from body cells. Foods like fruits and veggies supply lesser calories than what the body utilizes to metabolize them; thus, these foods are a great choice for weight loss.

Apart from being low in calorie and forcing the body to burn more calories to metabolize them, are such foods healthy? Critics of the negative calorie diet plan argue that a diet comprised of fewer food groups can offset the positive calorie energy reserves within the body. Low-calorie foods such as berries and broccoli could be rich in vitamins and minerals but also lack fats. Fats are important for weight loss because they make you full, avoiding instances of overeating. On the other hand, foods such as leafy greens and low-glycemic fruits are rich in antioxidants, enzymes, and other phytonutrients that facilitate weight loss. You also get fiber, which promotes fullness or satiety, and can help you fight binge eating.

This begs the question, how effective is the negative calorie diet? This book will seek to answer that question.

Thanks again for purchasing this book, I hope you enjoy it!

Table of Contents

Does The Negative Calorie Diet Work?

To promote optimum health, you need to consume sufficient amounts of food groups like carbs, proteins, fats, and water to keep the body hydrated. On the other hand, to lose weight, the recommendation is to create a calorie deficit so your body burns more calories than you consume.

Out of the total amount of calories you consume, the body uses 10-15 percent during the digestion process. Your metabolism also requires additional fuel to digest food compounds and absorb proteins, carbs, mineral fats, and other nutrients. The body gets energy from calories you take in; therefore, a lower calorie intake causes the body to burn stored fats for energy, which leads to weight loss.

When you eat negative calorie foods, you can eat these foods in unlimited quantities and still maintain a calorie deficit. Because these foods are satiating, you eat lesser carbs or processed foods. Research shows that foods such as processed carbs or other simple sugars often spike insulin levels, which in turn hinders fat metabolization in the body. Once you adopt a diet that has no sugar beverages, energy drinks, fries, or baked foods, you feel better and energetic.

A negative calorie diet eliminates food substances such as gluten, refined sugars, caffeine, and trans fats that hinder effective metabolism. These foods cause the accumulation of waste products and microorganism trigger agents. When you adopt a negative calorie diet, you consume foods such as fruits and veggies that are rich in antioxidants, fiber, and phytonutrients. Further, fruits and veggies offer detox benefits that facilitate cleansing and removal of toxins from the body. Most dieters on low-calorie foods normally report feeling clear headed and lighter within a few weeks of adopting the diet. The impressive thing about this diet plan is that you do not have to fast to detox or lose weight.

Role of Dietary Fiber

Another aspect of the negative calorie diet is that it comprises of high fiber foods such as fruits and veggies. The human body cannot properly utilize a section of the caloric energy from fiber; therefore, the body excretes what it cannot utilize. Low calorie fruits, as well as dark leafy green vegetables have a lower calorie density; they do not offer significant metabolizable calories. Such an effect also contributes to the negative calorie theory. A good example of such a scenario is that of celery where two large stalks of the veggie contain 20 calories and 2 grams of fiber or cellulose.

As opposed to animals like cows, we cannot digest cellulose and cannot absorb calories from it. Thus, when you consume celery, you do not add a significant amount of calories in your metabolism. Other leafy greens such as mustard greens, kales, and collard greens are also rich in fiber and are of higher nutritional value. Such foods have high nutrient density, promote satiety or fullness, are low in calorie, and have a high thermic effect.

What Is The Negative Calorie Effect?

The concept behind negative calorie foods is eating foods that have lower calories in order to create a calorie deficit in the body. The concept draws its basis on a theory called the negative calorie effect.

During the digestion process, the body needs additional fuel to breakdown and assimilate high proteins and fiber. When you eat negative calorie foods whether raw or slightly cooked, the body burns more calories during the breakdown process. Because of this reason, such foods have a greater thermic effect and thus help boost the basal metabolic rate and facilitate weight loss.

The actual thermic effect that you get varies depending on the type of food under question; for instance:

❖ Proteins have the highest thermic effect of about 30 percent

❖ Carbs follow with a relative thermic effect of around 15 percent

❖ Dietary fat has the lowest thermic effect of between 3-5 percent

Although veggies and fruits are the top most negative calorie foods, proteins have the highest thermic effect and thus would require more fuel to digest and metabolize.

So, why should you adopt the negative calorie diet?

Why Adopt Negative Calorie Diet And If The Diet Suits You

The most notable thing you stand to gain from adopting a negative calorie diet is weight loss in a scenario where you eat low calorie foods without monitoring your calorie intake. By adopting low calorie foods like fruits and veggies, you eliminate unhealthy foods and eat a diet that is more natural.

Eating natural foods allows you to shift your focus from the need to lose weight or feeling guilty about what you are eating, which allows you to concentrate on eating healthy foods. Once you start enjoying what you eat, you become motivated to stick to the program and thus lose weight easily. You no longer have to constantly resent your diet and crave for processed and unhealthy foods. Furthermore, the fiber from fruits and veggies keeps you fuller for longer, thus, you experience no diet crashes or feel the urge to cheat because you eat only when you are hungry.

Let us see a few benefits you stand to gain once you decide to adopt a negative calorie diet:

Optimal weight loss

As stated here, a negative calorie diet comprises of foods whose calorie level is much lower than what the body requires to metabolize them. For this mere reason, it is easy to shed some pounds and remain motivated to stick to the diet. In addition, the diet lowers cravings and fights the occasional hunger linked to high carb diet.

A negative calorie diet plan also allows you to eat fewer calories without feeling hungry and without calorie restrictions. This low calorie diet does not only help you lose body fat, it also helps you maintain body shape. Research shows that with negative calorie diet alone, it is possible to lose up to 2 pounds daily!

Helps manage insulin levels

A negative calorie diet helps you deal with sugar crashes linked to reduced sensitivity to insulin or insulin intolerance. Insulin has the ability to prevent the conversion of fat to energy in a process called lipolysis. Normal, high carb diets increase the level of insulin, which inhibits the lipolysis process. Diets low in calories and carbohydrates lower insulin levels and thus increase the rate of lipolysis. The process ensures that the body metabolizes fat for energy and prevents the breakdown of muscles for energy. In addition, the lowered insulin levels allows for the release of other beneficial hormones such as the growth hormone.

Reduced Risk of Sugar-Linked Diseases

A negative calorie diet does not comprise of high carb foods like starchy veggies, wheat products, complex carbs, and other calorie dense foods. Most of the high-carb foods we crave for also lead to various health problems; problems you can reverse within a few weeks of proper dieting. Common diseases linked to carbs or sugars include type II diabetes, non-alcoholic fatty acids, heart disease, teeth decay, and dental caries. Free sugars also play a key role in the development of conditions such as obesity, insulin resistance, high triglycerides, low HDL cholesterol, and cholesterol and metabolic syndrome.

A negative calorie diet plan does not have free sugar; thus, you can use it to restore your health and prevent worsening of the above stated conditions.

When you eat a high carb diet, the body breaks it down to glucose in the digestive tract and then absorbs it into the bloodstream. When glucose enters the bloodstream, it causes a spike in blood sugar. At this point, healthy people will produce insulin to regulate the sugar levels. However, some people have insulin resistance, and are unable to regulate blood sugar levels; this leads to the development of type 2 Diabetes.

After you switch to a negative calorie diet, you automatically lower the amount of available glucose in the blood, which reduces the need for insulin.

Ingredients like fruits and veggies are sources of minerals, vitamins, and fiber and can rev your metabolism.

Points to Note:

While you stand to benefit greatly from following the negative calorie diet, it is important to know some challenges of the diet and how to deal with them. Let us look at these challenges in the following section.

1. In some cases, getting back to a normal diet after being on the negative calorie diet can cause a few people to regain weight. Thus, you may want to be alternating between a negative calorie diet and incorporating healthy whole foods like lean protein, whole grains and fruits low in fructose.

2. Consuming only 2 food groups does not constitute a balanced diet. You can deal with this challenge by incorporating other food groups into your diet occasionally.

3. To some dieters, a restriction in calories can lead to the development of problems such as dizziness, menstrual irregularity, cold intolerance, edema, and fatigue. However, the good thing is once you get used to the diet, you stop experiencing some of these symptoms.

Before you can get started on the diet, it is important to know whether you are a suitable candidate to go on the diet. Let us find out more about this in the following chapter.

Is The Negative Calorie Diet Suitable For You

When talking about negative calories, understand that a calorie is a unit of energy and you can lose weight if you burn more calories than you consume. For instance, assume you consume a total of 1000 calories a day while your metabolism requires 1600 calories daily. Within 7 days, you will have lost around 3,500 calories equivalent to 1-pound of body weight.

When you adopt a negative calorie diet, you do not have to worry about how many calories you need to consume or burn. In theory, if you eat cucumbers, apples, celery, romaine lettuce and drink water in the right amounts, it is possible to lose weight without any extra effort.

While on the diet, you need to consume a wider variety of foods to supply your body with all nutrients it requires. Some nutritionists are of the view that relying solely on low-calorie foods can be both boring and unhealthy. For instance, the diet is not suitable for people extremely active such as athletes, bodybuilders or those engaged in extreme sports due to the low calorie intake.

Therefore, for active dieters, carb cycling is a much better choice as opposed to restricting your diet plan to low-calorie foods. The negative calorie diet also lacks sufficient proteins that helps in muscle growth and healthy omega 3 fatty acids that prevent cellular inflammation. Thus, if you want to build muscle, the negative calorie diet is not for you.

This diet is most suitable for people who are not active. However, this should not be a pass for you to exercise and engage in physical activity. Physical activity is great for you. Thus, whether you are trying to lose weight or not, ensure that you exercise, even if it is just going on walks or jogging.

Let us now look at what you eat while on a negative calorie diet.

What to Eat When On a Negative Calorie Diet

The bulk of foods in a negative calorie diet are fruits, veggies, and a few natural herbs and species. These foods, in addition to being low in calories, also comprise of surplus vitamins and minerals that speed up production of enzymes that help break down both the calories you consume and additional calories found in the digestive system.

Negative Calorie Veggies

Vegetables, especially the leafy green types are ideal sources of vitamins that boost your immune system and help to fight diseases. Although some vegetables are high in sugar, you can opt for organic vegetables because they have better nutritional value.

Veggies allowed in this diet plan should be high in nutrients and low on carbohydrates; these include dark and leafy greens such as spinach, broccoli, collard greens, celery, and kales. These are rich in high amounts of vitamin A and C, and folate, a mineral that helps in the synthesis and repair of DNA, as well as cell growth. You also obtain potassium, a vital electrolyte that helps in nerve transmission.

To benefit from essential minerals, ample fiber, and low calories, you can eat veggies as snacks, in a salad, or as a side dish. On the other hand, you can value other veggies such as onions, tomatoes, and garlic.

Let us see why specific veggies are beneficial when it comes to weight loss:

Asparagus

Asparagus is a negative calorie food that has 27 calories per cup, and can rev up your metabolism. Asparagus also has immense detox powers due to its high amino acid content that acts as a diuretic that helps excrete unwanted wastes from the body.

Eating asparagus regularly ensures you get an ample supply of copper, iron, protein, folate, and vitamins A, C, E, and K. You can enjoy the veggie as a raw natural tender shoot, or toss it in salads. You can also steam asparagus.

Turnips

These are definitely the skinnier cousin to potato, and can be a great source of vitamin C and fiber, in addition to being low in the glycemic index. The easiest way to turnips is to use them in stews and soups. However, you can also slice them raw into salads or use them in crudité due to their crunchy feeling. A cup of turnips has 36 calories.

Lettuce

With only 5 calories per cup, most varieties of lettuce such as romaine lettuce are rich in manganese, folic acid, and B vitamins. Manganese is important for monitoring blood sugar and boosts your immune function. When buying lettuce, choose the purple or green variety such as the red or green leaf because these are high in nutrients. To make a salad or snack from lettuce, just toss with zesty homemade vinaigrette.

Beets

A half cup of beets will supply you with 37 calories; thus, beets are low-carb veggies that are also rich in antioxidants that keep you cancer free. Beets are also rich in nutrients such as potassium, folate, fiber, and iron, and can incorporate well in most pasta dishes and salads. Go for the deep colored beets because they are rich in an antioxidant referred to as Betanin, an antioxidant known for its potency on improving health.

Arugula

This veggie has just 4 calories per cup and is low in fats. Arugula is high in fiber, vitamins A, C and K, and potassium powerhouse. The veggie can match well with your soups, salads, or other recipes where you need leafy greens.

Broccoli

Known as a superfood, broccoli is a negative calorie containing just 31 calories per cup; it is also a great source of minerals, fiber, and vitamins. Broccoli is rich in antioxidants that speed up your metabolism, help you shed weight, and fight breast and colon cancer. The active ingredient in broccoli is Sulforaphane, the ingredient that makes the veggie bitter. You can incorporate broccoli easily into dishes like casseroles, soups, sesame oil, mustard, or you can sauté it with oil for a better flavor.

Brussel Sprouts

Brussel sprouts are yet another negative calorie food that should be on your menu because of their low calorie levels of just 38 calories per cup.

Tomato

Every 100-gram serving of tomatoes you consume has 17 calories. Tomatoes are rich in lycopene that fights cancer, prevents heart disease, facilitates weight loss, and fights inflammation. Tomatoes also offer high amounts of vitamin C, which is good for the immune system, and calcium, which supports healthy teeth and bones. You can either cook tomatoes or eat them raw based on your liking; however, cooked tomatoes are much healthier.

Carrots

A 100-gram serving of carrots has 41 calories! For those with a sweet tooth, carrots can satisfy you and balance your blood sugar levels. A carrot has low sugar content and is rich in beta-carotene, a substance that reduces the risk of diabetes and controls blood sugar. If you are not intrigued by raw carrot sticks, you can slice carrots into thin strips, scatter them onto a baking sheet, add in olive oil, salt, and pepper, roast the carrot strips at 400°F for around 40 minutes, and enjoy.

Negative Calorie Fruits

Fruits such as tangerine, watermelon, strawberries, oranges, apricots, and grapes are negative calorie foods containing high amounts of fiber. The digestible fiber present in these fruits is important for the body in that it facilitates the breakdown of sugar found in fruit and other foods.

The body finds it harder to breakdown the fiber in fruits compared to how it digests other foods; thus, the body expends tons of calories digesting these fruits. Just like veggies, these fruits are rich in vitamin C that boosts immunity and function as antioxidant. Fruits like apricots and grapes are great sources of vitamin A that boosts vision and skin health.

Research has also revealed that citrus fruits can lower risks of stroke and other heart-related conditions. A study published in The Medical Journal noted that citrus fruits contain high amounts of flavonoids that correlate properly with lower risk of ischemic stroke. However, note that most fruits are not "zero calorie" and some contain excess fructose that may increase your calorie intake beyond what you can actually burn. You should eat fruits like bananas, figs, and avocados in moderation even though they are essential or rich in nutrients.

When on a negative calorie diet, consider the following fruits:

Strawberries

With just 49 calories per cup, strawberries are definitely a negative calorie food of choice. Sold in most groceries and supermarkets all year round, the fruit is rich in vitamin C and fat-fighting fiber. Studies reveal that vitamin C can make breathing easier especially if you suffer from exercise-induced asthma. A further research from Journal of Nutritional Biochemistry in 2014 established that eating ample strawberries helped dieters suffering from high cholesterol levels reduce risk of coronary problems.

A creative way to enjoy your delicious treat of strawberries is to prepare gazpacho soup by blending a cup of strawberries, 2 tablespoons red wine vinegar, and 2 tablespoons olive oil. Also add in 1/3 cup fresh mint or basil, 2 scallions, ½ cucumber, 1 red bell pepper, 3 medium-sized tomatoes and 1/3 cup water. To add taste, you can add in ¼ teaspoon black pepper and ½ teaspoon unprocessed salt. Process in a blender and then chill for about 2 hours then serve.

Honeydew Melon

Despite its sweet taste, the fruit has around 61 calories per cup; it has heart friendly potassium, as well as vitamin C.

You can eat honeydew melon wedges as a standalone snack, or use the fruit in salads, salsa, yoghurt, and smoothies. When buying honeydew melon, choose the one that feels heavy and with a waxy rind and avoid those with any soft spots. To make a quick salad, just toss cubed honeydew lemons with baby spinach, sliced cucumber, toasted almonds, crumbled feta cheese, and cherry tomatoes.

Blackberries

Most of the berries are negative calorie and blackberries are no exception with just 62 calories per cup. These berries are also rich in fiber; a cup of berries offers a whopping 8 grams of fiber and can satiate you for longer.

The great thing about fiber is that it slows digestion, makes you feel fuller, and helps you shed body fat. By eating blackberries, you also stand to benefit from vitamin K and various antioxidants that help fight disease-causing free radicals. Are you bored of mulching on berries as your afternoon snack? You can add 2 cups of blackberries, ½ teaspoon almond extract, 1-teaspoon cinnamon, 2 tablespoons maple syrup, and 1/3 cup water into a saucepan. Bring the mixture to a boil and then reduce the heat and simmer for 20 minutes. You can then dissolve 2 teaspoons cornstarch in a tablespoon water then stir into the mixture, and heat for 1 an additional minute.

Grapefruit

A grapefruit revs up your metabolism and aids in the fat breakdown process. The fruit is rich in vitamin C that can help you remain energized throughout the entire day and boosts your metabolism. Grape fruits also fight cancer and regulate cholesterol. Start your morning with a healthy bite of grape fruit. You can also use the fruit to replace sweet snacks.

Bear in mind that most fruits are higher in calorie compared to their vegetable counterparts.

Other Negative Calorie Foods

While fruits and veggies make up a large portion of the negative diet plan, some other foods you may want to try include:

Broth

A cup of broth has 10 calories and can come from a variety of ingredients such as seafood, miso, chicken, vegetable broth, or lean beef. Broth is both satiating and nourishing for your body, particularly if tossed in lean meat or dark leafy greens.

A great thing about broth is that you can consume it in high volumes, consume fewer calories, and be satiated. However, broth has a relative amount of sodium and thus may not be a great choice if you suffer from blood pressure problems.

Mushrooms

This delicacy only has 15 calorie per cup and comes in wide varieties such as shiitake, Portobello, maitake, and white button. All these diverse species of mushrooms contain a great amount of antioxidants that boost your immunity as you shed pounds. When you consume mushrooms, you also get vitamins and minerals like phosphorus, thiamin, copper, niacin, potassium, and fiber. Consider the shiitake mushroom because it boasts of anti-cancer properties.

Coffee

Whether consumed for breakfast or as an afternoon snack, coffee is a great choice of drink because it has zero or no calories. Once you drink coffee, it alters the levels of natural hormones that monitor hunger in the body. Coffee also reduces the risk of liver and colon cancer, type II diabetes, and Parkinson's disease.

For those wishing to lose weight, caffeine has been proven to facilitate faster metabolism and fat burning. Drinking coffee also inhibits insulin spike to facilitate fat metabolism. To make coffee effective for weight loss, ensure that you do not add sugar or milk.

Coconut oil

Fats and oils are not low calorie compared to veggies, but taking a few teaspoons of healthier oils like coconut oil can help you shed a few pounds. This oil serves as a potent source of Lauric acid, a heart healthy fatty acid that has antiviral and anti-bacterial properties. Because of these properties, coconut oil is a great choice for boosting the immune system; it does so by destroying various harmful bacteria and viruses. If you are trying to lose weight, coconut oil can help burn fat and clean up the body because of its ability to process long chain fatty acids. The acid present in coconut oil supports immune system in babies.

Let us now look at what you should not eat while on the low calorie diet.

Negative Calorie Diet Don'ts

A negative calorie diet does not allow a majority of high carb or sugary foods, but a few products could be beneficial if the energy required to digest them is higher than what they provide. However, you should avoid the following foods:

Sugars

Avoid sweet products, or any food substance that contains brown sugar, cane sugar, corn syrup, honey, or sucrose. Most packaged or processed foods are high in wheat and sugars and have high levels of carbs. In addition, avoid canned soups and stews because most contain hidden starchy thickeners.

Grains

Avoid a majority of grains and products made from grains because of their high carb content; you should not eat wheat flour, pasta, pancakes, cookies, and ordinary cakes. However, a few grains such as bulgur, soba noodles, teff, wheat bran, air popped popcorn, rice cakes, and sandwich thins are considered low calorie.

Sugary beverages

These include drinks such as juice, sodas, as well as alcohol. Juices come from concentrated sugar of the original fruit, while non-diet sodas contain large amounts of fructose. Avoid alcohol because it is a product of grain, which has high carb content. If you have to drink, look for low carb beers to ensure you only drink low calorie drinks.

Milk

Ordinary milk is rich in proteins and fats but high in the sugar, lactose. However, fermented milk products have less lactose since the bacteria used to ferment consumes up all the lactose. You can enjoy a few glasses of low-fat yoghurt.

How to Prepare Zero Calorie Meals

Foods such as leafy greens often lose essential nutrients once subjected to high heat; thus, you should know how to prepare them. The most recommended method for cooking these foods include steaming, grilling, and eating raw as a salad.

Steaming

This is a great cooking method for veggies that have a delicate flavor. This method of cooking facilitates the retainment of essential nutrients when you compare it to a cooking method such as boiling.

You can also steam foods such as broccoli, asparagus, cauliflower, and green beans. To add flavor, consider adding unprocessed salt such as Himalayan salt and a squeeze of lemon. In case you need to add an eastern flare to your meals, you can steam broccoli and then add in some diced garlic and white pepper.

Grilling

This cooking method is best for foods such as asparagus, zucchini, and summer squash, and works well alongside a light coating of olive oil or butter.

Make a Salad

A majority of veggies can comfortably fit in most salad recipes, and can work well as a power-packed breakfast or lunch. You can combine leafy green veggies, bell peppers, carrots, tomatoes, and then add a teaspoon of olive oil, chili, and black pepper. Do not include the commercial version of ranch dressing due to additives that interfere with effective metabolism. Consider adding in diced apricots, apples, strawberries or other healthy fruits to incorporate some natural sweetness.

Be aware that additives like common salt have sodium that is not good if you are dealing with high blood pressure. Choose any unprocessed salt preferably one with a reddish-brown tint as it contain 84 trace minerals. Such nutrients include calcium, iron, and potassium and can offer additional health benefits while on the negative calorie diet.

How to Successfully Adopt the Negative Calorie Diet

To achieve success as you adopt this diet:

Eat the right type of fiber

As stated here, fiber is a core pillar of this diet plan, and there are two types of fiber, soluble and insoluble. Soluble fiber comes from foods such as veggies and fruits such as citrus fruits, apples, and strawberries. This soluble fiber slows down digestion of foods, which regulates blood sugar and cholesterol levels.

On the other hand, insoluble fiber comes from carrots, cauliflower, turnips, Brussels sprouts, beets and cabbage. Insoluble fiber assists in excretion of toxic wastes through the intestines and stomach. It also monitors stomach acidity thus helping fight microbes that cause cancer.

Apart from controlling blood sugar level, fiber fights fat retention because it plays a role in the processing of dietary fat. Fiber attaches to dietary fat, which allows for its extraction from your body. Fiber also encourages satiety and sustains optimum energy level by slowing down the digestion process. You need to consume about 21-35 grams of fiber daily, and more if you are active. Slowly increase your fiber intake by 2-4 grams daily from consumption of veggies and fruits to avoid effects such as gas, cramping, and bloating.

Add protein shake to your meal

When on a negative calorie diet, your main sources of fuel are low calorie fruits and veggies. Remember that your body needs proteins because proteins facilitate general growth, repair of worn out cells, synthesis, and monitoring of hormones in the blood stream. If you find a sit-down protein breakfast hard to sustain, consider taking a protein bar or protein shake to rev your metabolism. Go for protein shakes high in protein, rich in calcium and fiber, low in added sugar, and with no hydrogenated oils.

Also, decide what time of day you detect an energy slump and complement that slump with protein intake. These times depends on your activity level, daily schedule, and choice of meals. Incorporate proteins into your diet by adding at least one protein food per negative calorie meal. Protein source can be part of your side dish or an appetizer. To eat protein items every 4 hours, carry your protein bite to the office to allow for easy snacking. A protein bite also maintains sufficient energy levels and prevents unhealthy snacks that hinder weight loss.

Eat enough vitamins

Vitamins support weight loss by strengthening your body cells, muscles, bones, and supplying the body with the required energy. Vitamins such as vitamin B help your body cells make protein, release energy, and to manufacture serotonin, an essential brain chemical. The rule of thumb is to get sufficient amounts of vitamin A, B, C and K from ingredients approved in this negative calorie diet. You can get vitamin B from leafy green veggies such as spinach broccoli.

Eat acidic foods

Acidic foods such as vinegar, lime, and lemon juice slow down your digestion and thus make you feel fuller for longer. Most of these foods are also low in calorie and can ease the monotony of eating fruits and veggies as your main staple. It is easy to incorporate acidic foods into your veggies and salads, or alternatively, use them in marinades.

Conclusion

Thank you again for purchasing this book!

I hope you have learnt about the negative calorie diet and you are excited to get started.

The next step is to start re-stocking your pantry with the negative calorie foods and slowly get rid of the foods that you should not be eating.

Thank you and good luck!

www.ingramcontent.com/pod-product-compliance
Lightning Source LLC
Chambersburg PA
CBHW062030280526
45787CB00005B/2268